ELIMI

THE GOAL OF AN ELIMINATION ... WE EAT THAT TRIGGER A FLARE OR NE... ...IES. THIS CAN BE PARTICULARLY HELPFUL WHEN SUFFERING FROM INTERSTITIAL CYSTITIS AS FOOD RELATED TRIGGERS ARE COMMON. THIS WORKBOOK IS MEANT TO GUIDE YOU THROUGH THE PROCESS OF ELIMINATION AND REINTRODUCTION OF FOODS THAT ARE COMMON IRRITANTS OR FOODS THAT ARE CONSUMED OFTEN AND BELEIVED TO BE POSSIBLE PROBLEM FOODS.

YOU'LL FIRST BE ASKED TO WRITE A LIST OF FOODS YOU WISH TO ELIMINATED, BASED ON YOUR PERSONAL NEEDS. FOR INTERSTITIAL CYSTITIS THERE ARE COMMON PROBLEM FOODS WHICH WILL BE LISTED ON THE FOLLOWING PAGES. ADD THE FOODS FROM THAT LIST THAT YOU CONSUME IN YOUR DIET AS WELL AS THE FOODS YOU CONSUME OFTEN. AS EACH PERSON IS UNIQUE, CERTAIN FOODS MAY BE A TRIGGER FOOD FOR ONE PERSON AND NOT ANOTHER.

START A DIET THAT REFRAINS FROM ALL FOODS ON YOUR TRIGGER LIST FOR FOUR WEEKS. DEPENDING ON YOUR PERSONAL SITUATION YOU MAY FIND THAT AFTER TWO OR THREE WEEKS YOUR FOOD RELATED FLARES HAVE SUBSIDED, YOU CAN BEGIN THE REINTRODUCTION PROCESS AT THIS TIME.

THE FOOD DIARY SECTION PROVIDES SPACE TO RECORD THE FOODS BEING REINRODUCED. IT IS RECOMMENDED TO DO THIS WITH ONE FOOD AT A TIME, OVER A THREE DAY PERIOD. START WITH A HALF PORTION ON DAY ONE, IF NO FLARES OCCUR THEN MOVE ONTO DAY TWO AND SO ON. IF YOU EXPEREINCE A FLARE KEEP THE FOOD ON YOUR TRIGGER FOOD LIST AND MOVE ON TO THE NEXT ITEM. MAKE SURE TO WRITE DOWN ANY NEGATIVE RESPONSES OR FLARES ALONG WITH THEIR SEVERITY. NOTE, SOME PEOPLE EXPERIENCE A FLARE TOWARDS FOODS AFTER 20 MINUTES WHILE OTHERS SAY IT CAN TAKE UP TO 4 HOURS. IF YOU WANT TO RETEST A PROBLEM ITEM, REPEAT THE SAME THREE DAY PROCESS.

SEE THE INFORMATION PAGES AT THE BACK OF THE BOOK FOR TIPS ON FLARE TYPES AND SELF CARE TO EASE FLARE SEVERITY.

MOST BOTHERSOME

THESE FOODS ARE REPORTED TO BE THE MOST LIKELY TO CAUSE A FLARE FOR PEOPLE WITH IC.

- COFFEE
- TEA
- SODA
- ALCOHOL
- CITRUS FRUITS AND JUICE
- CRANBERRY JUICE
- ARTIFICIAL SWEETNERS
- HOT PEPPERS
- SPICY FOODS
- MSG
- TOMATOES
- CHOCOLATE
- VITAMINS
- SUPPLEMENTS
- PICKLES
- SOY
- PROCESSED MEAT
- YOGURT
- KETCHUP
- SALAD DRESSINGS
- SOY SAUCE
- HORSERADISH
- CHILLI PEPPERS
- SAUERKRAUT
- MUSTARD
- VINEGAR

LEAST BOTHERSOME

THESE FOODS ARE REPORTED TO BE THE LEAST LIKELY TO CAUSE A FLARE FOR PEOPLE WITH IC.

- NON ACIDIC FRUITS
- AVOCADOA
- BEETS
- BROCCOLI
- POTATOES
- PEAS
- SPINACH
- COCONUT / OIL
- OATS
- RICE
- EGGS
- PEANUT BUTTER
- MEAT LIKE POULTRY, BEEF, LAMB
- MILK / CHEESE
- OLIVE OIL
- WATER
- POPCORN
- PRETZELS
- ALMONDS
- WHITE CHOCOLATE
- PARSLEY

- MINT
- GARLIC
- FENNEL
- DILL
- SAGE
- THYME
- VANILLA

TRIGGER FOODS

- .... REINTRODUCED ☐
- .... REINTRODUCED ☐
- .... REINTRODUCED ☐
- .... REINTRODUCED ☐
- .... REINTRODUCED ☐
- .... REINTRODUCED ☐
- .... REINTRODUCED ☐
- .... REINTRODUCED ☐
- .... REINTRODUCED ☐
- .... REINTRODUCED ☐
- .... REINTRODUCED ☐
- .... REINTRODUCED ☐
- .... REINTRODUCED ☐
- .... REINTRODUCED ☐
- .... REINTRODUCED ☐
- .... REINTRODUCED ☐
- .... REINTRODUCED ☐
- .... REINTRODUCED ☐

TRIGGER FOODS

- .... REINTRODUCED ☐
- .... REINTRODUCED ☐
- .... REINTRODUCED ☐
- .... REINTRODUCED ☐
- .... REINTRODUCED ☐
- .... REINTRODUCED ☐
- .... REINTRODUCED ☐
- .... REINTRODUCED ☐
- .... REINTRODUCED ☐
- .... REINTRODUCED ☐
- .... REINTRODUCED ☐
- .... REINTRODUCED ☐
- .... REINTRODUCED ☐
- .... REINTRODUCED ☐
- .... REINTRODUCED ☐
- .... REINTRODUCED ☐
- .... REINTRODUCED ☐

TRIGGER FOODS

- ....REINTRODUCED ☐
- ....REINTRODUCED ☐
- ....REINTRODUCED ☐
- ....REINTRODUCED ☐
- ....REINTRODUCED ☐
- ....REINTRODUCED ☐
- ....REINTRODUCED ☐
- ....REINTRODUCED ☐
- ....REINTRODUCED ☐
- ....REINTRODUCED ☐
- ....REINTRODUCED ☐
- ....REINTRODUCED ☐
- ....REINTRODUCED ☐
- ....REINTRODUCED ☐
- ....REINTRODUCED ☐
- ....REINTRODUCED ☐
- ....REINTRODUCED ☐
- ....REINTRODUCED ☐

TRIGGER FOODS

- ....REINTRODUCED ☐
- ....REINTRODUCED ☐
- ....REINTRODUCED ☐
- ....REINTRODUCED ☐
- ....REINTRODUCED ☐
- ....REINTRODUCED ☐
- ....REINTRODUCED ☐
- ....REINTRODUCED ☐
- ....REINTRODUCED ☐
- ....REINTRODUCED ☐
- ....REINTRODUCED ☐
- ....REINTRODUCED ☐
- ....REINTRODUCED ☐
- ....REINTRODUCED ☐
- ....REINTRODUCED ☐
- ....REINTRODUCED ☐

TRIGGER FOODS

- .... REINTRODUCED ☐
- .... REINTRODUCED ☐
- .... REINTRODUCED ☐
- .... REINTRODUCED ☐
- .... REINTRODUCED ☐
- .... REINTRODUCED ☐
- .... REINTRODUCED ☐
- .... REINTRODUCED ☐
- .... REINTRODUCED ☐
- .... REINTRODUCED ☐
- .... REINTRODUCED ☐
- .... REINTRODUCED ☐
- .... REINTRODUCED ☐
- .... REINTRODUCED ☐
- .... REINTRODUCED ☐
- .... REINTRODUCED ☐
- .... REINTRODUCED ☐

TRIGGER FOODS

- .... REINTRODUCED ☐
- .... REINTRODUCED ☐
- .... REINTRODUCED ☐
- .... REINTRODUCED ☐
- .... REINTRODUCED ☐
- .... REINTRODUCED ☐
- .... REINTRODUCED ☐
- .... REINTRODUCED ☐
- .... REINTRODUCED ☐
- .... REINTRODUCED ☐
- .... REINTRODUCED ☐
- .... REINTRODUCED ☐
- .... REINTRODUCED ☐
- .... REINTRODUCED ☐
- .... REINTRODUCED ☐
- .... REINTRODUCED ☐
- .... REINTRODUCED ☐

TRIGGER FOODS

- ....REINTRODUCED ☐
- ....REINTRODUCED ☐
- ....REINTRODUCED ☐
- ....REINTRODUCED ☐
- ....REINTRODUCED ☐
- ....REINTRODUCED ☐
- ....REINTRODUCED ☐
- ....REINTRODUCED ☐
- ....REINTRODUCED ☐
- ....REINTRODUCED ☐
- ....REINTRODUCED ☐
- ....REINTRODUCED ☐
- ....REINTRODUCED ☐
- ....REINTRODUCED ☐
- ....REINTRODUCED ☐
- ....REINTRODUCED ☐
- ....REINTRODUCED ☐

TRIGGER FOODS

- .... REINTRODUCED ☐
- .... REINTRODUCED ☐
- .... REINTRODUCED ☐
- .... REINTRODUCED ☐
- .... REINTRODUCED ☐
- .... REINTRODUCED ☐
- .... REINTRODUCED ☐
- .... REINTRODUCED ☐
- .... REINTRODUCED ☐
- .... REINTRODUCED ☐
- .... REINTRODUCED ☐
- .... REINTRODUCED ☐
- .... REINTRODUCED ☐
- .... REINTRODUCED ☐
- .... REINTRODUCED ☐
- .... REINTRODUCED ☐
- .... REINTRODUCED ☐

TRIGGER FOODS

- .... REINTRODUCED ☐
- .... REINTRODUCED ☐
- .... REINTRODUCED ☐
- .... REINTRODUCED ☐
- .... REINTRODUCED ☐
- .... REINTRODUCED ☐
- .... REINTRODUCED ☐
- .... REINTRODUCED ☐
- .... REINTRODUCED ☐
- .... REINTRODUCED ☐
- .... REINTRODUCED ☐
- .... REINTRODUCED ☐
- .... REINTRODUCED ☐
- .... REINTRODUCED ☐
- .... REINTRODUCED ☐
- .... REINTRODUCED ☐
- .... REINTRODUCED ☐
- .... REINTRODUCED ☐

TRIGGER FOODS

- .... REINTRODUCED ☐
- .... REINTRODUCED ☐
- .... REINTRODUCED ☐
- .... REINTRODUCED ☐
- .... REINTRODUCED ☐
- .... REINTRODUCED ☐
- .... REINTRODUCED ☐
- .... REINTRODUCED ☐
- .... REINTRODUCED ☐
- .... REINTRODUCED ☐
- .... REINTRODUCED ☐
- .... REINTRODUCED ☐
- .... REINTRODUCED ☐
- .... REINTRODUCED ☐
- .... REINTRODUCED ☐
- .... REINTRODUCED ☐
- .... REINTRODUCED ☐

FOOD DIARY

-FOOD: .... REINTRODUCED ☐

START DATE: ....

DAY ONE (1/2 PORTION)

FLARE: YES / NO   SEVERITY: ⚡⚡⚡⚡⚡

HOW YOU FELT AFTER EATING / SYMPTOMS:

....
....
....

DAY TWO (3/4 PORTION)

FLARE: YES / NO   SEVERITY: ⚡⚡⚡⚡⚡

HOW YOU FELT AFTER EATING / SYMPTOMS:

....
....
....

DAY THREE (1 PORTION)

FLARE: YES / NO   SEVERITY: ⚡⚡⚡⚡⚡

HOW YOU FELT AFTER EATING / SYMPTOMS:

....
....
....

FOOD DIARY

-FOOD: .... REINTRODUCED ☐

START DATE: ....

DAY ONE (1/2 PORTION)

FLARE: YES / NO   SEVERITY: ⚡ ⚡ ⚡ ⚡ ⚡

HOW YOU FELT AFTER EATING / SYMPTOMS:

....
....
....

DAY TWO (3/4 PORTION)

FLARE: YES / NO   SEVERITY: ⚡ ⚡ ⚡ ⚡ ⚡

HOW YOU FELT AFTER EATING / SYMPTOMS:

....
....
....

DAY THREE (1 PORTION)

FLARE: YES / NO   SEVERITY: ⚡ ⚡ ⚡ ⚡ ⚡

HOW YOU FELT AFTER EATING / SYMPTOMS:

....
....
....

FOOD DIARY

-FOOD: .... REINTRODUCED ☐

START DATE: ....

DAY ONE (1/2 PORTION)

FLARE: YES / NO   SEVERITY: ⚡ ⚡ ⚡ ⚡ ⚡

HOW YOU FELT AFTER EATING / SYMPTOMS:

....
....
....
....

DAY TWO (3/4 PORTION)

FLARE: YES / NO   SEVERITY: ⚡ ⚡ ⚡ ⚡ ⚡

HOW YOU FELT AFTER EATING / SYMPTOMS:

....
....
....
....

DAY THREE (1 PORTION)

FLARE: YES / NO   SEVERITY: ⚡ ⚡ ⚡ ⚡ ⚡

HOW YOU FELT AFTER EATING / SYMPTOMS:

....
....
....
....

FOOD DIARY

-FOOD: .... REINTRODUCED ☐

START DATE: ....

DAY ONE (1/2 PORTION)

FLARE: YES / NO   SEVERITY: ⚡ ⚡ ⚡ ⚡ ⚡

HOW YOU FELT AFTER EATING / SYMPTOMS:

....

....

....

....

DAY TWO (3/4 PORTION)

FLARE: YES / NO   SEVERITY: ⚡ ⚡ ⚡ ⚡ ⚡

HOW YOU FELT AFTER EATING / SYMPTOMS:

....

....

....

....

DAY THREE (1 PORTION)

FLARE: YES / NO   SEVERITY: ⚡ ⚡ ⚡ ⚡ ⚡

HOW YOU FELT AFTER EATING / SYMPTOMS:

....

....

....

....

FOOD DIARY

-FOOD: .... REINTRODUCED ☐
 START DATE: ....

DAY ONE (1/2 PORTION)

FLARE: YES / NO   SEVERITY: ⚡⚡⚡⚡⚡

HOW YOU FELT AFTER EATING / SYMPTOMS:

....
....
....

DAY TWO (3/4 PORTION)

FLARE: YES / NO   SEVERITY: ⚡⚡⚡⚡⚡

HOW YOU FELT AFTER EATING / SYMPTOMS:

....
....
....

DAY THREE (1 PORTION)

FLARE: YES / NO   SEVERITY: ⚡⚡⚡⚡⚡

HOW YOU FELT AFTER EATING / SYMPTOMS:

....
....
....

FOOD DIARY

-FOOD: .... REINTRODUCED ☐

START DATE: ....

DAY ONE (1/2 PORTION)

FLARE: YES / NO   SEVERITY: ⚡ ⚡ ⚡ ⚡ ⚡

HOW YOU FELT AFTER EATING / SYMPTOMS:

....
....
....
....

DAY TWO (3/4 PORTION)

FLARE: YES / NO   SEVERITY: ⚡ ⚡ ⚡ ⚡ ⚡

HOW YOU FELT AFTER EATING / SYMPTOMS:

....
....
....
....

DAY THREE (1 PORTION)

FLARE: YES / NO   SEVERITY: ⚡ ⚡ ⚡ ⚡ ⚡

HOW YOU FELT AFTER EATING / SYMPTOMS:

....
....
....
....

FOOD DIARY

-FOOD: .... REINTRODUCED ☐

START DATE: ....

DAY ONE (1/2 PORTION)

FLARE: YES / NO   SEVERITY: ⚡⚡⚡⚡⚡

HOW YOU FELT AFTER EATING / SYMPTOMS:

....

....

....

....

DAY TWO (3/4 PORTION)

FLARE: YES / NO   SEVERITY: ⚡⚡⚡⚡⚡

HOW YOU FELT AFTER EATING / SYMPTOMS:

....

....

....

....

DAY THREE (1 PORTION)

FLARE: YES / NO   SEVERITY: ⚡⚡⚡⚡⚡

HOW YOU FELT AFTER EATING / SYMPTOMS:

....

....

....

....

FOOD DIARY

-FOOD: .... REINTRODUCED ☐

START DATE: ....

DAY ONE (1/2 PORTION)

FLARE: YES / NO   SEVERITY: ⚡ ⚡ ⚡ ⚡ ⚡

HOW YOU FELT AFTER EATING / SYMPTOMS:

....
....
....
....

DAY TWO (3/4 PORTION)

FLARE: YES / NO   SEVERITY: ⚡ ⚡ ⚡ ⚡ ⚡

HOW YOU FELT AFTER EATING / SYMPTOMS:

....
....
....
....

DAY THREE (1 PORTION)

FLARE: YES / NO   SEVERITY: ⚡ ⚡ ⚡ ⚡ ⚡

HOW YOU FELT AFTER EATING / SYMPTOMS:

....
....
....
....

FOOD DIARY

-FOOD: .... REINTRODUCED ☐

START DATE: ....

DAY ONE (1/2 PORTION)

FLARE: YES / NO   SEVERITY: ⚡ ⚡ ⚡ ⚡ ⚡

HOW YOU FELT AFTER EATING / SYMPTOMS:

....
....
....

DAY TWO (3/4 PORTION)

FLARE: YES / NO   SEVERITY: ⚡ ⚡ ⚡ ⚡ ⚡

HOW YOU FELT AFTER EATING / SYMPTOMS:

....
....
....

DAY THREE (1 PORTION)

FLARE: YES / NO   SEVERITY: ⚡ ⚡ ⚡ ⚡ ⚡

HOW YOU FELT AFTER EATING / SYMPTOMS:

....
....
....

FOOD DIARY

FOOD: .... REINTRODUCED ☐

START DATE: ....

DAY ONE (1/2 PORTION)

FLARE: YES / NO   SEVERITY: ⚡ ⚡ ⚡ ⚡ ⚡

HOW YOU FELT AFTER EATING / SYMPTOMS:
....
....
....

DAY TWO (3/4 PORTION)

FLARE: YES / NO   SEVERITY: ⚡ ⚡ ⚡ ⚡ ⚡

HOW YOU FELT AFTER EATING / SYMPTOMS:
....
....
....

DAY THREE (1 PORTION)

FLARE: YES / NO   SEVERITY: ⚡ ⚡ ⚡ ⚡ ⚡

HOW YOU FELT AFTER EATING / SYMPTOMS:
....
....
....

FOOD DIARY

-FOOD: .... REINTRODUCED ☐

START DATE: ....

DAY ONE (1/2 PORTION)

FLARE: YES / NO   SEVERITY: ⚡⚡⚡⚡⚡

HOW YOU FELT AFTER EATING / SYMPTOMS:

....
....
....
....

DAY TWO (3/4 PORTION)

FLARE: YES / NO   SEVERITY: ⚡⚡⚡⚡⚡

HOW YOU FELT AFTER EATING / SYMPTOMS:

....
....
....
....

DAY THREE (1 PORTION)

FLARE: YES / NO   SEVERITY: ⚡⚡⚡⚡⚡

HOW YOU FELT AFTER EATING / SYMPTOMS:

....
....
....
....

FOOD DIARY

-FOOD: .... REINTRODUCED ☐

START DATE: ....

DAY ONE (1/2 PORTION)

FLARE: YES / NO   SEVERITY: ⚡ ⚡ ⚡ ⚡ ⚡

HOW YOU FELT AFTER EATING / SYMPTOMS:

....
....
....

DAY TWO (3/4 PORTION)

FLARE: YES / NO   SEVERITY: ⚡ ⚡ ⚡ ⚡ ⚡

HOW YOU FELT AFTER EATING / SYMPTOMS:

....
....
....

DAY THREE (1 PORTION)

FLARE: YES / NO   SEVERITY: ⚡ ⚡ ⚡ ⚡ ⚡

HOW YOU FELT AFTER EATING / SYMPTOMS:

....
....
....

FOOD DIARY

-FOOD: .... REINTRODUCED ☐

START DATE: ....

DAY ONE (1/2 PORTION)

FLARE: YES / NO   SEVERITY: ⚡⚡⚡⚡⚡

HOW YOU FELT AFTER EATING / SYMPTOMS:

....

....

....

DAY TWO (3/4 PORTION)

FLARE: YES / NO   SEVERITY: ⚡⚡⚡⚡⚡

HOW YOU FELT AFTER EATING / SYMPTOMS:

....

....

....

DAY THREE (1 PORTION)

FLARE: YES / NO   SEVERITY: ⚡⚡⚡⚡⚡

HOW YOU FELT AFTER EATING / SYMPTOMS:

....

....

....

FOOD DIARY

-FOOD: .... REINTRODUCED ☐

START DATE: ....

DAY ONE (1/2 PORTION)

FLARE: YES / NO   SEVERITY: ⚡ ⚡ ⚡ ⚡ ⚡

HOW YOU FELT AFTER EATING / SYMPTOMS:

....

....

....

DAY TWO (3/4 PORTION)

FLARE: YES / NO   SEVERITY: ⚡ ⚡ ⚡ ⚡ ⚡

HOW YOU FELT AFTER EATING / SYMPTOMS:

....

....

....

DAY THREE (1 PORTION)

FLARE: YES / NO   SEVERITY: ⚡ ⚡ ⚡ ⚡ ⚡

HOW YOU FELT AFTER EATING / SYMPTOMS:

....

....

....

FOOD DIARY

-FOOD: .... REINTRODUCED ☐

START DATE: ....

DAY ONE (1/2 PORTION)

FLARE: YES / NO   SEVERITY: ⚡ ⚡ ⚡ ⚡ ⚡

HOW YOU FELT AFTER EATING / SYMPTOMS:

....
....
....

DAY TWO (3/4 PORTION)

FLARE: YES / NO   SEVERITY: ⚡ ⚡ ⚡ ⚡ ⚡

HOW YOU FELT AFTER EATING / SYMPTOMS:

....
....
....

DAY THREE (1 PORTION)

FLARE: YES / NO   SEVERITY: ⚡ ⚡ ⚡ ⚡ ⚡

HOW YOU FELT AFTER EATING / SYMPTOMS:

....
....
....

FOOD DIARY

FOOD: .... REINTRODUCED ☐

START DATE: ....

DAY ONE (1/2 PORTION)

FLARE: YES / NO   SEVERITY: ⚡⚡⚡⚡⚡

HOW YOU FELT AFTER EATING / SYMPTOMS:

....
....
....

DAY TWO (3/4 PORTION)

FLARE: YES / NO   SEVERITY: ⚡⚡⚡⚡⚡

HOW YOU FELT AFTER EATING / SYMPTOMS:

....
....
....

DAY THREE (1 PORTION)

FLARE: YES / NO   SEVERITY: ⚡⚡⚡⚡⚡

HOW YOU FELT AFTER EATING / SYMPTOMS:

....
....
....

FOOD DIARY

-FOOD: .... REINTRODUCED ☐

START DATE: ....

DAY ONE (1/2 PORTION)

FLARE: YES / NO   SEVERITY: ⚡⚡⚡⚡⚡

HOW YOU FELT AFTER EATING / SYMPTOMS:

....

....

....

DAY TWO (3/4 PORTION)

FLARE: YES / NO   SEVERITY: ⚡⚡⚡⚡⚡

HOW YOU FELT AFTER EATING / SYMPTOMS:

....

....

....

DAY THREE (1 PORTION)

FLARE: YES / NO   SEVERITY: ⚡⚡⚡⚡⚡

HOW YOU FELT AFTER EATING / SYMPTOMS:

....

....

....

FOOD DIARY

-FOOD: .... REINTRODUCED ☐

START DATE: ....

DAY ONE (1/2 PORTION)

FLARE: YES / NO   SEVERITY: ⚡⚡⚡⚡⚡

HOW YOU FELT AFTER EATING / SYMPTOMS:
....
....
....

DAY TWO (3/4 PORTION)

FLARE: YES / NO   SEVERITY: ⚡⚡⚡⚡⚡

HOW YOU FELT AFTER EATING / SYMPTOMS:
....
....
....

DAY THREE (1 PORTION)

FLARE: YES / NO   SEVERITY: ⚡⚡⚡⚡⚡

HOW YOU FELT AFTER EATING / SYMPTOMS:
....
....
....

FOOD DIARY

-FOOD: .... REINTRODUCED ☐

START DATE: ....

DAY ONE (1/2 PORTION)

FLARE: YES / NO   SEVERITY: ⚡ ⚡ ⚡ ⚡ ⚡

HOW YOU FELT AFTER EATING / SYMPTOMS:

....

....

....

DAY TWO (3/4 PORTION)

FLARE: YES / NO   SEVERITY: ⚡ ⚡ ⚡ ⚡ ⚡

HOW YOU FELT AFTER EATING / SYMPTOMS:

....

....

....

DAY THREE (1 PORTION)

FLARE: YES / NO   SEVERITY: ⚡ ⚡ ⚡ ⚡ ⚡

HOW YOU FELT AFTER EATING / SYMPTOMS:

....

....

....

FOOD DIARY

FOOD: .... REINTRODUCED ☐

START DATE: ....

DAY ONE (1/2 PORTION)

FLARE: YES / NO   SEVERITY: ⚡⚡⚡⚡⚡

HOW YOU FELT AFTER EATING / SYMPTOMS:

DAY TWO (3/4 PORTION)

FLARE: YES / NO   SEVERITY: ⚡⚡⚡⚡⚡

HOW YOU FELT AFTER EATING / SYMPTOMS:

DAY THREE (1 PORTION)

FLARE: YES / NO   SEVERITY: ⚡⚡⚡⚡⚡

HOW YOU FELT AFTER EATING / SYMPTOMS:

FOOD DIARY

-FOOD: .... REINTRODUCED ☐

START DATE: ....

DAY ONE (1/2 PORTION)

FLARE: YES / NO   SEVERITY: ⚡⚡⚡⚡⚡

HOW YOU FELT AFTER EATING / SYMPTOMS:

....

....

....

DAY TWO (3/4 PORTION)

FLARE: YES / NO   SEVERITY: ⚡⚡⚡⚡⚡

HOW YOU FELT AFTER EATING / SYMPTOMS:

....

....

....

DAY THREE (1 PORTION)

FLARE: YES / NO   SEVERITY: ⚡⚡⚡⚡⚡

HOW YOU FELT AFTER EATING / SYMPTOMS:

....

....

....

FOOD DIARY

FOOD: .... REINTRODUCED ☐

START DATE: ....

DAY ONE (1/2 PORTION)

FLARE: YES / NO   SEVERITY: ⚡ ⚡ ⚡ ⚡ ⚡

HOW YOU FELT AFTER EATING / SYMPTOMS:

....
....
....
....

DAY TWO (3/4 PORTION)

FLARE: YES / NO   SEVERITY: ⚡ ⚡ ⚡ ⚡ ⚡

HOW YOU FELT AFTER EATING / SYMPTOMS:

....
....
....
....

DAY THREE (1 PORTION)

FLARE: YES / NO   SEVERITY: ⚡ ⚡ ⚡ ⚡ ⚡

HOW YOU FELT AFTER EATING / SYMPTOMS:

....
....
....
....

FOOD DIARY

-FOOD: .... REINTRODUCED ☐

START DATE: ....

DAY ONE (1/2 PORTION)

FLARE: YES / NO   SEVERITY: ⚡ ⚡ ⚡ ⚡ ⚡

HOW YOU FELT AFTER EATING / SYMPTOMS:

....

....

....

DAY TWO (3/4 PORTION)

FLARE: YES / NO   SEVERITY: ⚡ ⚡ ⚡ ⚡ ⚡

HOW YOU FELT AFTER EATING / SYMPTOMS:

....

....

....

DAY THREE (1 PORTION)

FLARE: YES / NO   SEVERITY: ⚡ ⚡ ⚡ ⚡ ⚡

HOW YOU FELT AFTER EATING / SYMPTOMS:

....

....

....

FOOD DIARY

FOOD: .... REINTRODUCED ☐

START DATE: ....

DAY ONE (1/2 PORTION)

FLARE: YES / NO   SEVERITY: ⚡⚡⚡⚡⚡

HOW YOU FELT AFTER EATING / SYMPTOMS:

....
....
....
....

DAY TWO (3/4 PORTION)

FLARE: YES / NO   SEVERITY: ⚡⚡⚡⚡⚡

HOW YOU FELT AFTER EATING / SYMPTOMS:

....
....
....
....

DAY THREE (1 PORTION)

FLARE: YES / NO   SEVERITY: ⚡⚡⚡⚡⚡

HOW YOU FELT AFTER EATING / SYMPTOMS:

....
....
....
....

FOOD DIARY

-FOOD: .... REINTRODUCED ☐

STARTDATE: ....

DAY ONE (1/2 PORTION)

FLARE: YES / NO　　　　　　　SEVERITY: ⚡ ⚡ ⚡ ⚡ ⚡

HOW YOU FELT AFTER EATING / SYMPTOMS:

....
....
....

DAY TWO (3/4 PORTION)

FLARE: YES / NO　　　　　　　SEVERITY: ⚡ ⚡ ⚡ ⚡ ⚡

HOW YOU FELT AFTER EATING / SYMPTOMS:

....
....
....

DAY THREE (1 PORTION)

FLARE: YES / NO　　　　　　　SEVERITY: ⚡ ⚡ ⚡ ⚡ ⚡

HOW YOU FELT AFTER EATING / SYMPTOMS:

....
....
....

FOOD DIARY

FOOD: .... REINTRODUCED ☐

START DATE: ....

DAY ONE (1/2 PORTION)

FLARE: YES / NO   SEVERITY: ⚡ ⚡ ⚡ ⚡ ⚡

HOW YOU FELT AFTER EATING / SYMPTOMS:

....

....

....

....

DAY TWO (3/4 PORTION)

FLARE: YES / NO   SEVERITY: ⚡ ⚡ ⚡ ⚡ ⚡

HOW YOU FELT AFTER EATING / SYMPTOMS:

....

....

....

....

DAY THREE (1 PORTION)

FLARE: YES / NO   SEVERITY: ⚡ ⚡ ⚡ ⚡ ⚡

HOW YOU FELT AFTER EATING / SYMPTOMS:

....

....

....

....

FOOD DIARY

-FOOD: .... REINTRODUCED ☐

 START DATE: ....

DAY ONE (1/2 PORTION)

FLARE: YES / NO   SEVERITY: ⚡ ⚡ ⚡ ⚡ ⚡

HOW YOU FELT AFTER EATING / SYMPTOMS:

....
....
....
....

DAY TWO (3/4 PORTION)

FLARE: YES / NO   SEVERITY: ⚡ ⚡ ⚡ ⚡ ⚡

HOW YOU FELT AFTER EATING / SYMPTOMS:

....
....
....
....

DAY THREE (1 PORTION)

FLARE: YES / NO   SEVERITY: ⚡ ⚡ ⚡ ⚡ ⚡

HOW YOU FELT AFTER EATING / SYMPTOMS:

....
....
....
....

FOOD DIARY

-FOOD: .... REINTRODUCED ☐

START DATE: ....

DAY ONE (1/2 PORTION)

FLARE: YES / NO   SEVERITY: ⚡ ⚡ ⚡ ⚡ ⚡

HOW YOU FELT AFTER EATING / SYMPTOMS:

....
....
....

DAY TWO (3/4 PORTION)

FLARE: YES / NO   SEVERITY: ⚡ ⚡ ⚡ ⚡ ⚡

HOW YOU FELT AFTER EATING / SYMPTOMS:

....
....
....

DAY THREE (1 PORTION)

FLARE: YES / NO   SEVERITY: ⚡ ⚡ ⚡ ⚡ ⚡

HOW YOU FELT AFTER EATING / SYMPTOMS:

....
....
....

FOOD DIARY

-FOOD: .... REINTRODUCED ☐

START DATE: ....

DAY ONE (1/2 PORTION)

FLARE: YES / NO					SEVERITY: ⚡⚡⚡⚡⚡

HOW YOU FELT AFTER EATING / SYMPTOMS:

....
....
....
....

DAY TWO (3/4 PORTION)

FLARE: YES / NO					SEVERITY: ⚡⚡⚡⚡⚡

HOW YOU FELT AFTER EATING / SYMPTOMS:

....
....
....
....

DAY THREE (1 PORTION)

FLARE: YES / NO					SEVERITY: ⚡⚡⚡⚡⚡

HOW YOU FELT AFTER EATING / SYMPTOMS:

....
....
....
....

FOOD DIARY

-FOOD: .... REINTRODUCED ☐

 START DATE: ....

DAY ONE (1/2 PORTION)

FLARE: YES / NO   SEVERITY: ⚡⚡⚡⚡⚡

HOW YOU FELT AFTER EATING / SYMPTOMS:

....
....
....
....

DAY TWO (3/4 PORTION)

FLARE: YES / NO   SEVERITY: ⚡⚡⚡⚡⚡

HOW YOU FELT AFTER EATING / SYMPTOMS:

....
....
....
....

DAY THREE (1 PORTION)

FLARE: YES / NO   SEVERITY: ⚡⚡⚡⚡⚡

HOW YOU FELT AFTER EATING / SYMPTOMS:

....
....
....
....

FOOD DIARY

-FOOD: .... REINTRODUCED ☐

START DATE: ....

DAY ONE (1/2 PORTION)

FLARE: YES / NO   SEVERITY: ⚡⚡⚡⚡⚡

HOW YOU FELT AFTER EATING / SYMPTOMS:

....
....
....

DAY TWO (3/4 PORTION)

FLARE: YES / NO   SEVERITY: ⚡⚡⚡⚡⚡

HOW YOU FELT AFTER EATING / SYMPTOMS:

....
....
....

DAY THREE (1 PORTION)

FLARE: YES / NO   SEVERITY: ⚡⚡⚡⚡⚡

HOW YOU FELT AFTER EATING / SYMPTOMS:

....
....
....

FOOD DIARY

FOOD: .... REINTRODUCED ☐

START DATE: ....

DAY ONE (1/2 PORTION)

FLARE: YES / NO   SEVERITY: ⚡⚡⚡⚡⚡

HOW YOU FELT AFTER EATING / SYMPTOMS:

....
....
....

DAY TWO (3/4 PORTION)

FLARE: YES / NO   SEVERITY: ⚡⚡⚡⚡⚡

HOW YOU FELT AFTER EATING / SYMPTOMS:

....
....
....

DAY THREE (1 PORTION)

FLARE: YES / NO   SEVERITY: ⚡⚡⚡⚡⚡

HOW YOU FELT AFTER EATING / SYMPTOMS:

....
....
....

FOOD DIARY

-FOOD: .... REINTRODUCED ☐

START DATE: ....

DAY ONE (1/2 PORTION)

FLARE: YES / NO   SEVERITY: ⚡ ⚡ ⚡ ⚡ ⚡

HOW YOU FELT AFTER EATING / SYMPTOMS:

....
....
....
....

DAY TWO (3/4 PORTION)

FLARE: YES / NO   SEVERITY: ⚡ ⚡ ⚡ ⚡ ⚡

HOW YOU FELT AFTER EATING / SYMPTOMS:

....
....
....
....

DAY THREE (1 PORTION)

FLARE: YES / NO   SEVERITY: ⚡ ⚡ ⚡ ⚡ ⚡

HOW YOU FELT AFTER EATING / SYMPTOMS:

....
....
....
....

FOOD DIARY

-FOOD: .... REINTRODUCED ☐

START DATE: ....

DAY ONE (1/2 PORTION)

FLARE: YES / NO   SEVERITY: ⚡⚡⚡⚡⚡

HOW YOU FELT AFTER EATING / SYMPTOMS:

....
....
....

DAY TWO (3/4 PORTION)

FLARE: YES / NO   SEVERITY: ⚡⚡⚡⚡⚡

HOW YOU FELT AFTER EATING / SYMPTOMS:

....
....
....

DAY THREE (1 PORTION)

FLARE: YES / NO   SEVERITY: ⚡⚡⚡⚡⚡

HOW YOU FELT AFTER EATING / SYMPTOMS:

....
....
....

FOOD DIARY

-FOOD: .... REINTRODUCED ☐

START DATE: ....

DAY ONE (1/2 PORTION)

FLARE: YES / NO   SEVERITY: ⚡⚡⚡⚡⚡

HOW YOU FELT AFTER EATING / SYMPTOMS:

....
....
....

DAY TWO (3/4 PORTION)

FLARE: YES / NO   SEVERITY: ⚡⚡⚡⚡⚡

HOW YOU FELT AFTER EATING / SYMPTOMS:

....
....
....

DAY THREE (1 PORTION)

FLARE: YES / NO   SEVERITY: ⚡⚡⚡⚡⚡

HOW YOU FELT AFTER EATING / SYMPTOMS:

....
....
....

FOOD DIARY

FOOD: .... REINTRODUCED ☐

START DATE: ....

DAY ONE (1/2 PORTION)

FLARE: YES / NO   SEVERITY: ⚡ ⚡ ⚡ ⚡ ⚡

HOW YOU FELT AFTER EATING / SYMPTOMS:

....
....
....

DAY TWO (3/4 PORTION)

FLARE: YES / NO   SEVERITY: ⚡ ⚡ ⚡ ⚡ ⚡

HOW YOU FELT AFTER EATING / SYMPTOMS:

....
....
....

DAY THREE (1 PORTION)

FLARE: YES / NO   SEVERITY: ⚡ ⚡ ⚡ ⚡ ⚡

HOW YOU FELT AFTER EATING / SYMPTOMS:

....
....
....

FOOD DIARY

-FOOD: .... REINTRODUCED ☐

START DATE: ....

DAY ONE (1/2 PORTION)

FLARE: YES / NO   SEVERITY: ⚡⚡⚡⚡⚡

HOW YOU FELT AFTER EATING / SYMPTOMS:

....
....
....

DAY TWO (3/4 PORTION)

FLARE: YES / NO   SEVERITY: ⚡⚡⚡⚡⚡

HOW YOU FELT AFTER EATING / SYMPTOMS:

....
....
....

DAY THREE (1 PORTION)

FLARE: YES / NO   SEVERITY: ⚡⚡⚡⚡⚡

HOW YOU FELT AFTER EATING / SYMPTOMS:

....
....
....

FOOD DIARY

FOOD: .... REINTRODUCED ☐

START DATE: ....

DAY ONE (1/2 PORTION)

FLARE: YES / NO   SEVERITY: ⚡⚡⚡⚡⚡

HOW YOU FELT AFTER EATING / SYMPTOMS:

....
....
....

DAY TWO (3/4 PORTION)

FLARE: YES / NO   SEVERITY: ⚡⚡⚡⚡⚡

HOW YOU FELT AFTER EATING / SYMPTOMS:

....
....
....

DAY THREE (1 PORTION)

FLARE: YES / NO   SEVERITY: ⚡⚡⚡⚡⚡

HOW YOU FELT AFTER EATING / SYMPTOMS:

....
....
....

FOOD DIARY

-FOOD: .... REINTRODUCED ☐

START DATE: ....

DAY ONE (1/2 PORTION)

FLARE: YES / NO　　　　　　　　SEVERITY: ⚡⚡⚡⚡⚡

HOW YOU FELT AFTER EATING / SYMPTOMS:

....
....
....

DAY TWO (3/4 PORTION)

FLARE: YES / NO　　　　　　　　SEVERITY: ⚡⚡⚡⚡⚡

HOW YOU FELT AFTER EATING / SYMPTOMS:

....
....
....

DAY THREE (1 PORTION)

FLARE: YES / NO　　　　　　　　SEVERITY: ⚡⚡⚡⚡⚡

HOW YOU FELT AFTER EATING / SYMPTOMS:

....
....
....

FOOD DIARY

FOOD: .... REINTRODUCED ☐

START DATE: ....

DAY ONE (1/2 PORTION)

FLARE: YES / NO   SEVERITY: ⚡⚡⚡⚡⚡

HOW YOU FELT AFTER EATING / SYMPTOMS:

....

....

....

DAY TWO (3/4 PORTION)

FLARE: YES / NO   SEVERITY: ⚡⚡⚡⚡⚡

HOW YOU FELT AFTER EATING / SYMPTOMS:

....

....

....

DAY THREE (1 PORTION)

FLARE: YES / NO   SEVERITY: ⚡⚡⚡⚡⚡

HOW YOU FELT AFTER EATING / SYMPTOMS:

....

....

....

FOOD DIARY

-FOOD: .... REINTRODUCED ☐

START DATE: ....

DAY ONE (1/2 PORTION)

FLARE: YES / NO   SEVERITY: ⚡⚡⚡⚡⚡

HOW YOU FELT AFTER EATING / SYMPTOMS:

....
....
....

DAY TWO (3/4 PORTION)

FLARE: YES / NO   SEVERITY: ⚡⚡⚡⚡⚡

HOW YOU FELT AFTER EATING / SYMPTOMS:

....
....
....

DAY THREE (1 PORTION)

FLARE: YES / NO   SEVERITY: ⚡⚡⚡⚡⚡

HOW YOU FELT AFTER EATING / SYMPTOMS:

....
....
....

FOOD DIARY

FOOD: .... REINTRODUCED ☐

START DATE: ....

DAY ONE (1/2 PORTION)

FLARE: YES / NO   SEVERITY: ⚡⚡⚡⚡⚡

HOW YOU FELT AFTER EATING / SYMPTOMS:

....
....
....

DAY TWO (3/4 PORTION)

FLARE: YES / NO   SEVERITY: ⚡⚡⚡⚡⚡

HOW YOU FELT AFTER EATING / SYMPTOMS:

....
....
....

DAY THREE (1 PORTION)

FLARE: YES / NO   SEVERITY: ⚡⚡⚡⚡⚡

HOW YOU FELT AFTER EATING / SYMPTOMS:

....
....
....

FOOD DIARY

-FOOD: .... REINTRODUCED ☐

　STA RT DATE: ....

DAY ONE (1/2 PORTION)

FLARE: YES / NO　　　　　　　SEVERITY: ⚡⚡⚡⚡⚡

HOW YOU FELT AFTER EATING / SYMPTOMS:

....
....
....
....

DAY TWO (3/4 PORTION)

FLARE: YES / NO　　　　　　　SEVERITY: ⚡⚡⚡⚡⚡

HOW YOU FELT AFTER EATING / SYMPTOMS:

....
....
....
....

DAY THREE (1 PORTION)

FLARE: YES / NO　　　　　　　SEVERITY: ⚡⚡⚡⚡⚡

HOW YOU FELT AFTER EATING / SYMPTOMS:

....
....
....
....

FOOD DIARY

-FOOD: .... REINTRODUCED ☐

START DATE: ....

DAY ONE (1/2 PORTION)

FLARE: YES / NO   SEVERITY: ⚡⚡⚡⚡⚡

HOW YOU FELT AFTER EATING / SYMPTOMS:

....
....
....
....

DAY TWO (3/4 PORTION)

FLARE: YES / NO   SEVERITY: ⚡⚡⚡⚡⚡

HOW YOU FELT AFTER EATING / SYMPTOMS:

....
....
....
....

DAY THREE (1 PORTION)

FLARE: YES / NO   SEVERITY: ⚡⚡⚡⚡⚡

HOW YOU FELT AFTER EATING / SYMPTOMS:

....
....
....
....

FOOD DIARY

-FOOD: .... REINTRODUCED ☐

START DATE: ....

DAY ONE (1/2 PORTION)

FLARE: YES / NO   SEVERITY: ⚡⚡⚡⚡⚡

HOW YOU FELT AFTER EATING / SYMPTOMS:

....
....
....
....

DAY TWO (3/4 PORTION)

FLARE: YES / NO   SEVERITY: ⚡⚡⚡⚡⚡

HOW YOU FELT AFTER EATING / SYMPTOMS:

....
....
....
....

DAY THREE (1 PORTION)

FLARE: YES / NO   SEVERITY: ⚡⚡⚡⚡⚡

HOW YOU FELT AFTER EATING / SYMPTOMS:

....
....
....
....

FOOD DIARY

-FOOD: .... REINTRODUCED ☐

START DATE: ....

DAY ONE (1/2 PORTION)

FLARE: YES / NO   SEVERITY: ⚡ ⚡ ⚡ ⚡ ⚡

HOW YOU FELT AFTER EATING / SYMPTOMS:

....

....

....

DAY TWO (3/4 PORTION)

FLARE: YES / NO   SEVERITY: ⚡ ⚡ ⚡ ⚡ ⚡

HOW YOU FELT AFTER EATING / SYMPTOMS:

....

....

....

DAY THREE (1 PORTION)

FLARE: YES / NO   SEVERITY: ⚡ ⚡ ⚡ ⚡ ⚡

HOW YOU FELT AFTER EATING / SYMPTOMS:

....

....

....

FOOD DIARY

-FOOD: .... REINTRODUCED ☐

START DATE: ....

DAY ONE (1/2 PORTION)

FLARE: YES / NO   SEVERITY: ⚡⚡⚡⚡⚡

HOW YOU FELT AFTER EATING / SYMPTOMS:

....

....

....

DAY TWO (3/4 PORTION)

FLARE: YES / NO   SEVERITY: ⚡⚡⚡⚡⚡

HOW YOU FELT AFTER EATING / SYMPTOMS:

....

....

....

DAY THREE (1 PORTION)

FLARE: YES / NO   SEVERITY: ⚡⚡⚡⚡⚡

HOW YOU FELT AFTER EATING / SYMPTOMS:

....

....

....

FOOD DIARY

FOOD: .... REINTRODUCED ☐

START DATE: ....

DAY ONE (1/2 PORTION)

FLARE: YES / NO   SEVERITY: ⚡ ⚡ ⚡ ⚡ ⚡

HOW YOU FELT AFTER EATING / SYMPTOMS:

....
....
....
....

DAY TWO (3/4 PORTION)

FLARE: YES / NO   SEVERITY: ⚡ ⚡ ⚡ ⚡ ⚡

HOW YOU FELT AFTER EATING / SYMPTOMS:

....
....
....
....

DAY THREE (1 PORTION)

FLARE: YES / NO   SEVERITY: ⚡ ⚡ ⚡ ⚡ ⚡

HOW YOU FELT AFTER EATING / SYMPTOMS:

....
....
....
....

FOOD DIARY

-FOOD: .... REINTRODUCED ☐

START DATE: ....

DAY ONE (1/2 PORTION)

FLARE: YES / NO   SEVERITY: ⚡⚡⚡⚡⚡

HOW YOU FELT AFTER EATING / SYMPTOMS:

....
....
....

DAY TWO (3/4 PORTION)

FLARE: YES / NO   SEVERITY: ⚡⚡⚡⚡⚡

HOW YOU FELT AFTER EATING / SYMPTOMS:

....
....
....

DAY THREE (1 PORTION)

FLARE: YES / NO   SEVERITY: ⚡⚡⚡⚡⚡

HOW YOU FELT AFTER EATING / SYMPTOMS:

....
....
....

FOOD DIARY

FOOD: .... REINTRODUCED ☐

START DATE: ....

DAY ONE (1/2 PORTION)

FLARE: YES / NO   SEVERITY: ⚡⚡⚡⚡⚡

HOW YOU FELT AFTER EATING / SYMPTOMS:

....
....
....

DAY TWO (3/4 PORTION)

FLARE: YES / NO   SEVERITY: ⚡⚡⚡⚡⚡

HOW YOU FELT AFTER EATING / SYMPTOMS:

....
....
....

DAY THREE (1 PORTION)

FLARE: YES / NO   SEVERITY: ⚡⚡⚡⚡⚡

HOW YOU FELT AFTER EATING / SYMPTOMS:

....
....
....

FOOD DIARY

-FOOD: .... REINTRODUCED ☐

START DATE: ....

DAY ONE (1/2 PORTION)

FLARE: YES / NO   SEVERITY: ⚡⚡⚡⚡⚡

HOW YOU FELT AFTER EATING / SYMPTOMS:

....
....
....

DAY TWO (3/4 PORTION)

FLARE: YES / NO   SEVERITY: ⚡⚡⚡⚡⚡

HOW YOU FELT AFTER EATING / SYMPTOMS:

....
....
....

DAY THREE (1 PORTION)

FLARE: YES / NO   SEVERITY: ⚡⚡⚡⚡⚡

HOW YOU FELT AFTER EATING / SYMPTOMS:

....
....
....

FOOD DIARY

-FOOD: .... REINTRODUCED ☐

START DATE: ....

DAY ONE (1/2 PORTION)

FLARE: YES / NO   SEVERITY: ⚡⚡⚡⚡⚡

HOW YOU FELT AFTER EATING / SYMPTOMS:
....
....
....
....

DAY TWO (3/4 PORTION)

FLARE: YES / NO   SEVERITY: ⚡⚡⚡⚡⚡

HOW YOU FELT AFTER EATING / SYMPTOMS:
....
....
....
....

DAY THREE (1 PORTION)

FLARE: YES / NO   SEVERITY: ⚡⚡⚡⚡⚡

HOW YOU FELT AFTER EATING / SYMPTOMS:
....
....
....
....

FOOD DIARY

FOOD: .... REINTRODUCED ☐

START DATE: ....

DAY ONE (1/2 PORTION)

FLARE: YES / NO   SEVERITY: ⚡⚡⚡⚡⚡

HOW YOU FELT AFTER EATING / SYMPTOMS: ....

....

....

....

DAY TWO (3/4 PORTION)

FLARE: YES / NO   SEVERITY: ⚡⚡⚡⚡⚡

HOW YOU FELT AFTER EATING / SYMPTOMS:

....

....

....

DAY THREE (1 PORTION)

FLARE: YES / NO   SEVERITY: ⚡⚡⚡⚡⚡

HOW YOU FELT AFTER EATING / SYMPTOMS:

....

....

....

FOOD DIARY

FOOD: .... REINTRODUCED ☐

START DATE: ....

DAY ONE (1/2 PORTION)

FLARE: YES / NO   SEVERITY: ⚡⚡⚡⚡⚡

HOW YOU FELT AFTER EATING / SYMPTOMS:

....
....
....

DAY TWO (3/4 PORTION)

FLARE: YES / NO   SEVERITY: ⚡⚡⚡⚡⚡

HOW YOU FELT AFTER EATING / SYMPTOMS:

....
....
....

DAY THREE (1 PORTION)

FLARE: YES / NO   SEVERITY: ⚡⚡⚡⚡⚡

HOW YOU FELT AFTER EATING / SYMPTOMS:

....
....
....

FOOD DIARY

-FOOD: .... REINTRODUCED ☐

START DATE: ....

DAY ONE (1/2 PORTION)

FLARE: YES / NO   SEVERITY: ⚡⚡⚡⚡⚡

HOW YOU FELT AFTER EATING / SYMPTOMS:
....
....
....

DAY TWO (3/4 PORTION)

FLARE: YES / NO   SEVERITY: ⚡⚡⚡⚡⚡

HOW YOU FELT AFTER EATING / SYMPTOMS:
....
....
....

DAY THREE (1 PORTION)

FLARE: YES / NO   SEVERITY: ⚡⚡⚡⚡⚡

HOW YOU FELT AFTER EATING / SYMPTOMS:
....
....
....

FOOD DIARY

-FOOD: .... REINTRODUCED ☐

START DATE: ....

DAY ONE (1/2 PORTION)

FLARE: YES / NO   SEVERITY: ⚡⚡⚡⚡⚡

HOW YOU FELT AFTER EATING / SYMPTOMS:

....

....

....

DAY TWO (3/4 PORTION)

FLARE: YES / NO   SEVERITY: ⚡⚡⚡⚡⚡

HOW YOU FELT AFTER EATING / SYMPTOMS:

....

....

....

DAY THREE (1 PORTION)

FLARE: YES / NO   SEVERITY: ⚡⚡⚡⚡⚡

HOW YOU FELT AFTER EATING / SYMPTOMS:

....

....

....

FOOD DIARY

-FOOD: .... REINTRODUCED ☐

START DATE: ....

DAY ONE (1/2 PORTION)

FLARE: YES / NO   SEVERITY: ⚡⚡⚡⚡⚡

HOW YOU FELT AFTER EATING / SYMPTOMS:

....

....

....

DAY TWO (3/4 PORTION)

FLARE: YES / NO   SEVERITY: ⚡⚡⚡⚡⚡

HOW YOU FELT AFTER EATING / SYMPTOMS:

....

....

....

DAY THREE (1 PORTION)

FLARE: YES / NO   SEVERITY: ⚡⚡⚡⚡⚡

HOW YOU FELT AFTER EATING / SYMPTOMS:

....

....

....

FOOD DIARY

-FOOD: .... REINTRODUCED ☐

START DATE: ....

DAY ONE (1/2 PORTION)

FLARE: YES / NO   SEVERITY: ⚡⚡⚡⚡⚡

HOW YOU FELT AFTER EATING / SYMPTOMS:

....
....
....
....

DAY TWO (3/4 PORTION)

FLARE: YES / NO   SEVERITY: ⚡⚡⚡⚡⚡

HOW YOU FELT AFTER EATING / SYMPTOMS:

....
....
....
....

DAY THREE (1 PORTION)

FLARE: YES / NO   SEVERITY: ⚡⚡⚡⚡⚡

HOW YOU FELT AFTER EATING / SYMPTOMS:

....
....
....
....

FOOD DIARY

-FOOD: .... REINTRODUCED ☐

START DATE: ....

DAY ONE (1/2 PORTION)

FLARE: YES / NO   SEVERITY: ⚡⚡⚡⚡⚡

HOW YOU FELT AFTER EATING / SYMPTOMS:

....
....
....

DAY TWO (3/4 PORTION)

FLARE: YES / NO   SEVERITY: ⚡⚡⚡⚡⚡

HOW YOU FELT AFTER EATING / SYMPTOMS:

....
....
....

DAY THREE (1 PORTION)

FLARE: YES / NO   SEVERITY: ⚡⚡⚡⚡⚡

HOW YOU FELT AFTER EATING / SYMPTOMS:

....
....
....

FOOD DIARY

-FOOD: .... REINTRODUCED ☐

START DATE: ....

DAY ONE (1/2 PORTION)

FLARE: YES / NO   SEVERITY: ⚡⚡⚡⚡⚡

HOW YOU FELT AFTER EATING / SYMPTOMS:

....
....
....

DAY TWO (3/4 PORTION)

FLARE: YES / NO   SEVERITY: ⚡⚡⚡⚡⚡

HOW YOU FELT AFTER EATING / SYMPTOMS:

....
....
....

DAY THREE (1 PORTION)

FLARE: YES / NO   SEVERITY: ⚡⚡⚡⚡⚡

HOW YOU FELT AFTER EATING / SYMPTOMS:

....
....
....

FOOD DIARY

-FOOD: .... REINTRODUCED ☐

START DATE: ....

DAY ONE (1/2 PORTION)

FLARE: YES / NO   SEVERITY: ⚡ ⚡ ⚡ ⚡ ⚡

HOW YOU FELT AFTER EATING / SYMPTOMS:

....
....
....

DAY TWO (3/4 PORTION)

FLARE: YES / NO   SEVERITY: ⚡ ⚡ ⚡ ⚡ ⚡

HOW YOU FELT AFTER EATING / SYMPTOMS:

....
....
....

DAY THREE (1 PORTION)

FLARE: YES / NO   SEVERITY: ⚡ ⚡ ⚡ ⚡ ⚡

HOW YOU FELT AFTER EATING / SYMPTOMS:

....
....
....

FOOD DIARY

-FOOD: .... REINTRODUCED ☐

START DATE: ....

DAY ONE (1/2 PORTION)

FLARE: YES / NO 　　　　　　SEVERITY: ⚡⚡⚡⚡⚡

HOW YOU FELT AFTER EATING / SYMPTOMS:

....

....

....

DAY TWO (3/4 PORTION)

FLARE: YES / NO 　　　　　　SEVERITY: ⚡⚡⚡⚡⚡

HOW YOU FELT AFTER EATING / SYMPTOMS:

....

....

....

DAY THREE (1 PORTION)

FLARE: YES / NO 　　　　　　SEVERITY: ⚡⚡⚡⚡⚡

HOW YOU FELT AFTER EATING / SYMPTOMS:

....

....

....

FOOD DIARY

FOOD: .... REINTRODUCED ☐

START DATE: ....

DAY ONE (1/2 PORTION)

FLARE: YES / NO   SEVERITY: ⚡⚡⚡⚡⚡

HOW YOU FELT AFTER EATING / SYMPTOMS:

....

....

....

DAY TWO (3/4 PORTION)

FLARE: YES / NO   SEVERITY: ⚡⚡⚡⚡⚡

HOW YOU FELT AFTER EATING / SYMPTOMS:

....

....

....

DAY THREE (1 PORTION)

FLARE: YES / NO   SEVERITY: ⚡⚡⚡⚡⚡

HOW YOU FELT AFTER EATING / SYMPTOMS:

....

....

....

FOOD DIARY

-FOOD: .... REINTRODUCED ☐
 START DATE: ....

DAY ONE (1/2 PORTION)

FLARE: YES / NO   SEVERITY: ⚡⚡⚡⚡⚡

HOW YOU FELT AFTER EATING / SYMPTOMS:
....
....
....

DAY TWO (3/4 PORTION)

FLARE: YES / NO   SEVERITY: ⚡⚡⚡⚡⚡

HOW YOU FELT AFTER EATING / SYMPTOMS:
....
....
....

DAY THREE (1 PORTION)

FLARE: YES / NO   SEVERITY: ⚡⚡⚡⚡⚡

HOW YOU FELT AFTER EATING / SYMPTOMS:
....
....
....

FOOD DIARY

-FOOD: .... REINTRODUCED ☐

STARTDATE: ....

DAY ONE (1/2 PORTION)

FLARE: YES / NO　　　　　　　　SEVERITY: ⚡⚡⚡⚡⚡

HOW YOU FELT AFTER EATING / SYMPTOMS:

....
....
....

DAY TWO (3/4 PORTION)

FLARE: YES / NO　　　　　　　　SEVERITY: ⚡⚡⚡⚡⚡

HOW YOU FELT AFTER EATING / SYMPTOMS:

....
....
....

DAY THREE (1 PORTION)

FLARE: YES / NO　　　　　　　　SEVERITY: ⚡⚡⚡⚡⚡

HOW YOU FELT AFTER EATING / SYMPTOMS:

....
....
....

FOOD DIARY

-FOOD: .... REINTRODUCED ☐

START DATE: ....

DAY ONE (1/2 PORTION)

FLARE: YES / NO   SEVERITY: ⚡ ⚡ ⚡ ⚡ ⚡

HOW YOU FELT AFTER EATING / SYMPTOMS:

....

....

....

DAY TWO (3/4 PORTION)

FLARE: YES / NO   SEVERITY: ⚡ ⚡ ⚡ ⚡ ⚡

HOW YOU FELT AFTER EATING / SYMPTOMS:

....

....

....

DAY THREE (1 PORTION)

FLARE: YES / NO   SEVERITY: ⚡ ⚡ ⚡ ⚡ ⚡

HOW YOU FELT AFTER EATING / SYMPTOMS:

....

....

....

FOOD DIARY

-FOOD: .... REINTRODUCED ☐

STARTDATE: ....

DAY ONE (1/2 PORTION)

FLARE: YES / NO   SEVERITY: ⚡⚡⚡⚡⚡

HOW YOU FELT AFTER EATING / SYMPTOMS:

....
....
....

DAY TWO (3/4 PORTION)

FLARE: YES / NO   SEVERITY: ⚡⚡⚡⚡⚡

HOW YOU FELT AFTER EATING / SYMPTOMS:

....
....
....

DAY THREE (1 PORTION)

FLARE: YES / NO   SEVERITY: ⚡⚡⚡⚡⚡

HOW YOU FELT AFTER EATING / SYMPTOMS:

....
....
....

FOOD DIARY

-FOOD: .... REINTRODUCED ☐

START DATE: ....

DAY ONE (1/2 PORTION)

FLARE: YES / NO   SEVERITY: ⚡⚡⚡⚡⚡

HOW YOU FELT AFTER EATING / SYMPTOMS:

....
....
....

DAY TWO (3/4 PORTION)

FLARE: YES / NO   SEVERITY: ⚡⚡⚡⚡⚡

HOW YOU FELT AFTER EATING / SYMPTOMS:

....
....
....

DAY THREE (1 PORTION)

FLARE: YES / NO   SEVERITY: ⚡⚡⚡⚡⚡

HOW YOU FELT AFTER EATING / SYMPTOMS:

....
....
....

FOOD DIARY

-FOOD: .... REINTRODUCED ☐

START DATE: ....

DAY ONE (1/2 PORTION)

FLARE: YES / NO 　　　　　SEVERITY: ⚡⚡⚡⚡⚡

HOW YOU FELT AFTER EATING / SYMPTOMS:

....
....
....

DAY TWO (3/4 PORTION)

FLARE: YES / NO 　　　　　SEVERITY: ⚡⚡⚡⚡⚡

HOW YOU FELT AFTER EATING / SYMPTOMS:

....
....
....

DAY THREE (1 PORTION)

FLARE: YES / NO 　　　　　SEVERITY: ⚡⚡⚡⚡⚡

HOW YOU FELT AFTER EATING / SYMPTOMS:

....
....
....

FOOD DIARY

-FOOD: .... REINTRODUCED ☐

START DATE: ....

DAY ONE (1/2 PORTION)

FLARE: YES / NO   SEVERITY: ⚡⚡⚡⚡⚡

HOW YOU FELT AFTER EATING / SYMPTOMS:

....

....

....

DAY TWO (3/4 PORTION)

FLARE: YES / NO   SEVERITY: ⚡⚡⚡⚡⚡

HOW YOU FELT AFTER EATING / SYMPTOMS:

....

....

....

DAY THREE (1 PORTION)

FLARE: YES / NO   SEVERITY: ⚡⚡⚡⚡⚡

HOW YOU FELT AFTER EATING / SYMPTOMS:

....

....

....

FOOD DIARY

-FOOD: .... REINTRODUCED ☐

START DATE: ....

DAY ONE (1/2 PORTION)

FLARE: YES / NO　　　　　　　　SEVERITY: ⚡ ⚡ ⚡ ⚡ ⚡

HOW YOU FELT AFTER EATING / SYMPTOMS:

....

....

....

DAY TWO (3/4 PORTION)

FLARE: YES / NO　　　　　　　　SEVERITY: ⚡ ⚡ ⚡ ⚡ ⚡

HOW YOU FELT AFTER EATING / SYMPTOMS:

....

....

....

DAY THREE (1 PORTION)

FLARE: YES / NO　　　　　　　　SEVERITY: ⚡ ⚡ ⚡ ⚡ ⚡

HOW YOU FELT AFTER EATING / SYMPTOMS:

....

....

....

FOOD DIARY

FOOD: .... REINTRODUCED ☐

START DATE: ....

DAY ONE (1/2 PORTION)

FLARE: YES / NO   SEVERITY: ⚡ ⚡ ⚡ ⚡ ⚡

HOW YOU FELT AFTER EATING / SYMPTOMS:

....
....
....

DAY TWO (3/4 PORTION)

FLARE: YES / NO   SEVERITY: ⚡ ⚡ ⚡ ⚡ ⚡

HOW YOU FELT AFTER EATING / SYMPTOMS:

....
....
....

DAY THREE (1 PORTION)

FLARE: YES / NO   SEVERITY: ⚡ ⚡ ⚡ ⚡ ⚡

HOW YOU FELT AFTER EATING / SYMPTOMS:

....
....
....

FOOD DIARY

FOOD: .... REINTRODUCED ☐

START DATE: ....

DAY ONE (1/2 PORTION)

FLARE: YES / NO   SEVERITY: ⚡⚡⚡⚡⚡

HOW YOU FELT AFTER EATING / SYMPTOMS:

....

....

....

DAY TWO (3/4 PORTION)

FLARE: YES / NO   SEVERITY: ⚡⚡⚡⚡⚡

HOW YOU FELT AFTER EATING / SYMPTOMS:

....

....

....

DAY THREE (1 PORTION)

FLARE: YES / NO   SEVERITY: ⚡⚡⚡⚡⚡

HOW YOU FELT AFTER EATING / SYMPTOMS:

....

....

....

FOOD DIARY

-FOOD: .... REINTRODUCED ☐

START DATE: ....

DAY ONE (1/2 PORTION)

FLARE: YES / NO   SEVERITY: ⚡⚡⚡⚡⚡

HOW YOU FELT AFTER EATING / SYMPTOMS:

....
....
....

DAY TWO (3/4 PORTION)

FLARE: YES / NO   SEVERITY: ⚡⚡⚡⚡⚡

HOW YOU FELT AFTER EATING / SYMPTOMS:

....
....
....

DAY THREE (1 PORTION)

FLARE: YES / NO   SEVERITY: ⚡⚡⚡⚡⚡

HOW YOU FELT AFTER EATING / SYMPTOMS:

....
....
....

FOOD DIARY

-FOOD: .... REINTRODUCED ☐

START DATE: ....

DAY ONE (1/2 PORTION)

FLARE: YES / NO   SEVERITY: ⚡⚡⚡⚡⚡

HOW YOU FELT AFTER EATING / SYMPTOMS:

....

....

....

DAY TWO (3/4 PORTION)

FLARE: YES / NO   SEVERITY: ⚡⚡⚡⚡⚡

HOW YOU FELT AFTER EATING / SYMPTOMS:

....

....

....

DAY THREE (1 PORTION)

FLARE: YES / NO   SEVERITY: ⚡⚡⚡⚡⚡

HOW YOU FELT AFTER EATING / SYMPTOMS:

....

....

....

FOOD DIARY

-FOOD: .... REINTRODUCED ☐

START DATE: ....

DAY ONE (1/2 PORTION)

FLARE: YES / NO   SEVERITY: ⚡ ⚡ ⚡ ⚡ ⚡

HOW YOU FELT AFTER EATING / SYMPTOMS:

....

....

....

DAY TWO (3/4 PORTION)

FLARE: YES / NO   SEVERITY: ⚡ ⚡ ⚡ ⚡ ⚡

HOW YOU FELT AFTER EATING / SYMPTOMS:

....

....

....

DAY THREE (1 PORTION)

FLARE: YES / NO   SEVERITY: ⚡ ⚡ ⚡ ⚡ ⚡

HOW YOU FELT AFTER EATING / SYMPTOMS:

....

....

....

FOOD DIARY

-FOOD: .... REINTRODUCED ☐

START DATE: ....

DAY ONE (1/2 PORTION)

FLARE: YES / NO   SEVERITY: ⚡ ⚡ ⚡ ⚡ ⚡

HOW YOU FELT AFTER EATING / SYMPTOMS:

....
....
....

DAY TWO (3/4 PORTION)

FLARE: YES / NO   SEVERITY: ⚡ ⚡ ⚡ ⚡ ⚡

HOW YOU FELT AFTER EATING / SYMPTOMS:

....
....
....

DAY THREE (1 PORTION)

FLARE: YES / NO   SEVERITY: ⚡ ⚡ ⚡ ⚡ ⚡

HOW YOU FELT AFTER EATING / SYMPTOMS:

....
....
....

FOOD DIARY

-FOOD: .... REINTRODUCED ☐

START DATE: ....

DAY ONE (1/2 PORTION)

FLARE: YES / NO   SEVERITY: ⚡ ⚡ ⚡ ⚡ ⚡

HOW YOU FELT AFTER EATING / SYMPTOMS:

....

....

....

DAY TWO (3/4 PORTION)

FLARE: YES / NO   SEVERITY: ⚡ ⚡ ⚡ ⚡ ⚡

HOW YOU FELT AFTER EATING / SYMPTOMS:

....

....

....

DAY THREE (1 PORTION)

FLARE: YES / NO   SEVERITY: ⚡ ⚡ ⚡ ⚡ ⚡

HOW YOU FELT AFTER EATING / SYMPTOMS:

....

....

....

FOOD DIARY

-FOOD: .... REINTRODUCED ☐

STArT DATE: ....

DAY ONE (1/2 PORTION)

FLARE: YES / NO   SEVERITY: ⚡⚡⚡⚡⚡

HOW YOU FELT AFTER EATING / SYMPTOMS:
....
....
....

DAY TWO (3/4 PORTION)

FLARE: YES / NO   SEVERITY: ⚡⚡⚡⚡⚡

HOW YOU FELT AFTER EATING / SYMPTOMS:
....
....
....

DAY THREE (1 PORTION)

FLARE: YES / NO   SEVERITY: ⚡⚡⚡⚡⚡

HOW YOU FELT AFTER EATING / SYMPTOMS:
....
....
....

FOOD DIARY

FOOD: .... REINTRODUCED ☐

START DATE: ....

DAY ONE (1/2 PORTION)

FLARE: YES / NO   SEVERITY: ⚡⚡⚡⚡⚡

HOW YOU FELT AFTER EATING / SYMPTOMS:

....
....
....

DAY TWO (3/4 PORTION)

FLARE: YES / NO   SEVERITY: ⚡⚡⚡⚡⚡

HOW YOU FELT AFTER EATING / SYMPTOMS:

....
....
....

DAY THREE (1 PORTION)

FLARE: YES / NO   SEVERITY: ⚡⚡⚡⚡⚡

HOW YOU FELT AFTER EATING / SYMPTOMS:

....
....
....

FOOD DIARY

FOOD: .... REINTRODUCED ☐

START DATE: ....

DAY ONE (1/2 PORTION)

FLARE: YES / NO   SEVERITY: ⚡⚡⚡⚡⚡

HOW YOU FELT AFTER EATING / SYMPTOMS:

....

....

....

DAY TWO (3/4 PORTION)

FLARE: YES / NO   SEVERITY: ⚡⚡⚡⚡⚡

HOW YOU FELT AFTER EATING / SYMPTOMS:

....

....

....

DAY THREE (1 PORTION)

FLARE: YES / NO   SEVERITY: ⚡⚡⚡⚡⚡

HOW YOU FELT AFTER EATING / SYMPTOMS:

....

....

....

FOOD DIARY

-FOOD: .... REINTRODUCED ☐

START DATE: ....

DAY ONE (1/2 PORTION)

FLARE: YES / NO　　　　　　　SEVERITY: ⚡⚡⚡⚡⚡

HOW YOU FELT AFTER EATING / SYMPTOMS:

....

....

....

DAY TWO (3/4 PORTION)

FLARE: YES / NO　　　　　　　SEVERITY: ⚡⚡⚡⚡⚡

HOW YOU FELT AFTER EATING / SYMPTOMS:

....

....

....

DAY THREE (1 PORTION)

FLARE: YES / NO　　　　　　　SEVERITY: ⚡⚡⚡⚡⚡

HOW YOU FELT AFTER EATING / SYMPTOMS:

....

....

....

FOOD DIARY

-FOOD: .... REINTRODUCED ☐

START DATE: ....

DAY ONE (1/2 PORTION)

FLARE: YES / NO   SEVERITY: ⚡⚡⚡⚡⚡

HOW YOU FELT AFTER EATING / SYMPTOMS:

....

....

....

DAY TWO (3/4 PORTION)

FLARE: YES / NO   SEVERITY: ⚡⚡⚡⚡⚡

HOW YOU FELT AFTER EATING / SYMPTOMS:

....

....

....

DAY THREE (1 PORTION)

FLARE: YES / NO   SEVERITY: ⚡⚡⚡⚡⚡

HOW YOU FELT AFTER EATING / SYMPTOMS:

....

....

....

FOOD DIARY

-FOOD: .... REINTRODUCED ☐

START DATE: ....

DAY ONE (1/2 PORTION)

FLARE: YES / NO   SEVERITY: ⚡⚡⚡⚡⚡

HOW YOU FELT AFTER EATING / SYMPTOMS:

....
....
....

DAY TWO (3/4 PORTION)

FLARE: YES / NO   SEVERITY: ⚡⚡⚡⚡⚡

HOW YOU FELT AFTER EATING / SYMPTOMS:

....
....
....

DAY THREE (1 PORTION)

FLARE: YES / NO   SEVERITY: ⚡⚡⚡⚡⚡

HOW YOU FELT AFTER EATING / SYMPTOMS:

....
....
....

FOOD DIARY

-FOOD: .... REINTRODUCED ☐

START DATE: ....

DAY ONE (1/2 PORTION)

FLARE: YES / NO   SEVERITY: ⚡⚡⚡⚡⚡

HOW YOU FELT AFTER EATING / SYMPTOMS:

....

....

....

DAY TWO (3/4 PORTION)

FLARE: YES / NO   SEVERITY: ⚡⚡⚡⚡⚡

HOW YOU FELT AFTER EATING / SYMPTOMS:

....

....

....

DAY THREE (1 PORTION)

FLARE: YES / NO   SEVERITY: ⚡⚡⚡⚡⚡

HOW YOU FELT AFTER EATING / SYMPTOMS:

....

....

....

FOOD DIARY

-FOOD: .... REINTRODUCED ☐

START DATE: ....

DAY ONE (1/2 PORTION)

FLARE: YES / NO   SEVERITY: ⚡⚡⚡⚡⚡

HOW YOU FELT AFTER EATING / SYMPTOMS:

....
....
....

DAY TWO (3/4 PORTION)

FLARE: YES / NO   SEVERITY: ⚡⚡⚡⚡⚡

HOW YOU FELT AFTER EATING / SYMPTOMS:

....
....
....

DAY THREE (1 PORTION)

FLARE: YES / NO   SEVERITY: ⚡⚡⚡⚡⚡

HOW YOU FELT AFTER EATING / SYMPTOMS:

....
....
....

FOOD DIARY

-FOOD: .... REINTRODUCED ☐

STARTDATE: ....

DAY ONE (1/2 PORTION)

FLARE: YES / NO   SEVERITY: ⚡⚡⚡⚡⚡

HOW YOU FELT AFTER EATING / SYMPTOMS:
....
....
....

DAY TWO (3/4 PORTION)

FLARE: YES / NO   SEVERITY: ⚡⚡⚡⚡⚡

HOW YOU FELT AFTER EATING / SYMPTOMS:
....
....
....

DAY THREE (1 PORTION)

FLARE: YES / NO   SEVERITY: ⚡⚡⚡⚡⚡

HOW YOU FELT AFTER EATING / SYMPTOMS:
....
....
....

FOOD DIARY

-FOOD: .... REINTRODUCED ☐

START DATE: ....

DAY ONE (1/2 PORTION)

FLARE: YES / NO   SEVERITY: ⚡⚡⚡⚡⚡

HOW YOU FELT AFTER EATING / SYMPTOMS:

....
....
....

DAY TWO (3/4 PORTION)

FLARE: YES / NO   SEVERITY: ⚡⚡⚡⚡⚡

HOW YOU FELT AFTER EATING / SYMPTOMS:

....
....
....

DAY THREE (1 PORTION)

FLARE: YES / NO   SEVERITY: ⚡⚡⚡⚡⚡

HOW YOU FELT AFTER EATING / SYMPTOMS:

....
....
....

FOOD DIARY

-FOOD: .... REINTRODUCED ☐

START DATE: ....

DAY ONE (1/2 PORTION)

FLARE: YES / NO   SEVERITY: ⚡⚡⚡⚡⚡

HOW YOU FELT AFTER EATING / SYMPTOMS:

....

....

....

DAY TWO (3/4 PORTION)

FLARE: YES / NO   SEVERITY: ⚡⚡⚡⚡⚡

HOW YOU FELT AFTER EATING / SYMPTOMS:

....

....

....

DAY THREE (1 PORTION)

FLARE: YES / NO   SEVERITY: ⚡⚡⚡⚡⚡

HOW YOU FELT AFTER EATING / SYMPTOMS:

....

....

....

FOOD DIARY

-FOOD: .... REINTRODUCED ☐

START DATE: ....

DAY ONE (1/2 PORTION)

FLARE: YES / NO   SEVERITY: ⚡⚡⚡⚡⚡

HOW YOU FELT AFTER EATING / SYMPTOMS:

....
....
....

DAY TWO (3/4 PORTION)

FLARE: YES / NO   SEVERITY: ⚡⚡⚡⚡⚡

HOW YOU FELT AFTER EATING / SYMPTOMS:

....
....
....

DAY THREE (1 PORTION)

FLARE: YES / NO   SEVERITY: ⚡⚡⚡⚡⚡

HOW YOU FELT AFTER EATING / SYMPTOMS:

....
....
....

FOOD DIARY

-FOOD: .... REINTRODUCED ☐

START DATE: ....

DAY ONE (1/2 PORTION)

FLARE: YES / NO   SEVERITY: ⚡ ⚡ ⚡ ⚡ ⚡

HOW YOU FELT AFTER EATING / SYMPTOMS:

....
....
....

DAY TWO (3/4 PORTION)

FLARE: YES / NO   SEVERITY: ⚡ ⚡ ⚡ ⚡ ⚡

HOW YOU FELT AFTER EATING / SYMPTOMS:

....
....
....

DAY THREE (1 PORTION)

FLARE: YES / NO   SEVERITY: ⚡ ⚡ ⚡ ⚡ ⚡

HOW YOU FELT AFTER EATING / SYMPTOMS:

....
....
....

FOOD DIARY

-FOOD: .... REINTRODUCED ☐

START DATE: ....

DAY ONE (1/2 PORTION)

FLARE: YES / NO   SEVERITY: ⚡⚡⚡⚡⚡

HOW YOU FELT AFTER EATING / SYMPTOMS:

....
....
....

DAY TWO (3/4 PORTION)

FLARE: YES / NO   SEVERITY: ⚡⚡⚡⚡⚡

HOW YOU FELT AFTER EATING / SYMPTOMS:

....
....
....

DAY THREE (1 PORTION)

FLARE: YES / NO   SEVERITY: ⚡⚡⚡⚡⚡

HOW YOU FELT AFTER EATING / SYMPTOMS:

....
....
....

FOOD DIARY

FOOD: .... REINTRODUCED ☐

START DATE: ....

DAY ONE (1/2 PORTION)

FLARE: YES / NO   SEVERITY: ⚡⚡⚡⚡⚡

HOW YOU FELT AFTER EATING / SYMPTOMS:

....
....
....

DAY TWO (3/4 PORTION)

FLARE: YES / NO   SEVERITY: ⚡⚡⚡⚡⚡

HOW YOU FELT AFTER EATING / SYMPTOMS:

....
....
....

DAY THREE (1 PORTION)

FLARE: YES / NO   SEVERITY: ⚡⚡⚡⚡⚡

HOW YOU FELT AFTER EATING / SYMPTOMS:

....
....
....

FOOD DIARY

-FOOD: .... REINTRODUCED ☐

START DATE: ....

DAY ONE (1/2 PORTION)

FLARE: YES / NO   SEVERITY: ⚡ ⚡ ⚡ ⚡ ⚡

HOW YOU FELT AFTER EATING / SYMPTOMS:

....
....
....

DAY TWO (3/4 PORTION)

FLARE: YES / NO   SEVERITY: ⚡ ⚡ ⚡ ⚡ ⚡

HOW YOU FELT AFTER EATING / SYMPTOMS:

....
....
....

DAY THREE (1 PORTION)

FLARE: YES / NO   SEVERITY: ⚡ ⚡ ⚡ ⚡ ⚡

HOW YOU FELT AFTER EATING / SYMPTOMS:

....
....
....

FOOD DIARY

-FOOD: .... REINTRODUCED ☐

STAR T DATE: ....

DAY ONE (1/2 PORTION)

FLARE: YES / NO   SEVERITY: ⚡⚡⚡⚡⚡

HOW YOU FELT AFTER EATING / SYMPTOMS:

....
....
....

DAY TWO (3/4 PORTION)

FLARE: YES / NO   SEVERITY: ⚡⚡⚡⚡⚡

HOW YOU FELT AFTER EATING / SYMPTOMS:

....
....
....

DAY THREE (1 PORTION)

FLARE: YES / NO   SEVERITY: ⚡⚡⚡⚡⚡

HOW YOU FELT AFTER EATING / SYMPTOMS:

....
....
....

FOOD DIARY

-FOOD: .... REINTRODUCED ☐

START DATE: ....

DAY ONE (1/2 PORTION)

FLARE: YES / NO   SEVERITY: ⚡ ⚡ ⚡ ⚡ ⚡

HOW YOU FELT AFTER EATING / SYMPTOMS:

....
....
....
....

DAY TWO (3/4 PORTION)

FLARE: YES / NO   SEVERITY: ⚡ ⚡ ⚡ ⚡ ⚡

HOW YOU FELT AFTER EATING / SYMPTOMS:

....
....
....
....

DAY THREE (1 PORTION)

FLARE: YES / NO   SEVERITY: ⚡ ⚡ ⚡ ⚡ ⚡

HOW YOU FELT AFTER EATING / SYMPTOMS:

....
....
....
....

FOOD DIARY

-FOOD: .... REINTRODUCED ☐
START DATE: ....

DAY ONE (1/2 PORTION)

FLARE: YES / NO   SEVERITY: ⚡⚡⚡⚡⚡

HOW YOU FELT AFTER EATING / SYMPTOMS:

....
....
....

DAY TWO (3/4 PORTION)

FLARE: YES / NO   SEVERITY: ⚡⚡⚡⚡⚡

HOW YOU FELT AFTER EATING / SYMPTOMS:

....
....
....

DAY THREE (1 PORTION)

FLARE: YES / NO   SEVERITY: ⚡⚡⚡⚡⚡

HOW YOU FELT AFTER EATING / SYMPTOMS:

....
....
....

FOOD DIARY

-FOOD: .... REINTRODUCED ☐

START DATE: ....

DAY ONE (1/2 PORTION)

FLARE: YES / NO   SEVERITY: ⚡⚡⚡⚡⚡

HOW YOU FELT AFTER EATING / SYMPTOMS:

....
....
....

DAY TWO (3/4 PORTION)

FLARE: YES / NO   SEVERITY: ⚡⚡⚡⚡⚡

HOW YOU FELT AFTER EATING / SYMPTOMS:

....
....
....

DAY THREE (1 PORTION)

FLARE: YES / NO   SEVERITY: ⚡⚡⚡⚡⚡

HOW YOU FELT AFTER EATING / SYMPTOMS:

....
....
....

FOOD DIARY

-FOOD: .... REINTRODUCED ☐

START DATE: ....

DAY ONE (1/2 PORTION)

FLARE: YES / NO   SEVERITY: ⚡⚡⚡⚡⚡

HOW YOU FELT AFTER EATING / SYMPTOMS:

....

....

....

DAY TWO (3/4 PORTION)

FLARE: YES / NO   SEVERITY: ⚡⚡⚡⚡⚡

HOW YOU FELT AFTER EATING / SYMPTOMS:

....

....

....

DAY THREE (1 PORTION)

FLARE: YES / NO   SEVERITY: ⚡⚡⚡⚡⚡

HOW YOU FELT AFTER EATING / SYMPTOMS:

....

....

....

FOOD DIARY

-FOOD: .... REINTRODUCED ☐

START DATE: ....

DAY ONE (1/2 PORTION)

FLARE: YES / NO   SEVERITY: ⚡⚡⚡⚡⚡

HOW YOU FELT AFTER EATING / SYMPTOMS:

....
....
....

DAY TWO (3/4 PORTION)

FLARE: YES / NO   SEVERITY: ⚡⚡⚡⚡⚡

HOW YOU FELT AFTER EATING / SYMPTOMS:

....
....
....

DAY THREE (1 PORTION)

FLARE: YES / NO   SEVERITY: ⚡⚡⚡⚡⚡

HOW YOU FELT AFTER EATING / SYMPTOMS:

....
....
....

FOOD DIARY

FOOD: .... REINTRODUCED ☐
START DATE: ....

DAY ONE (1/2 PORTION)

FLARE: YES / NO   SEVERITY: ⚡⚡⚡⚡⚡

HOW YOU FELT AFTER EATING / SYMPTOMS:
....
....
....

DAY TWO (3/4 PORTION)

FLARE: YES / NO   SEVERITY: ⚡⚡⚡⚡⚡

HOW YOU FELT AFTER EATING / SYMPTOMS:
....
....
....

DAY THREE (1 PORTION)

FLARE: YES / NO   SEVERITY: ⚡⚡⚡⚡⚡

HOW YOU FELT AFTER EATING / SYMPTOMS:
....
....
....

FOOD DIARY

-FOOD: .... REINTRODUCED ☐

START DATE: ....

DAY ONE (1/2 PORTION)

FLARE: YES / NO   SEVERITY: ⚡⚡⚡⚡⚡

HOW YOU FELT AFTER EATING / SYMPTOMS:

....
....
....

DAY TWO (3/4 PORTION)

FLARE: YES / NO   SEVERITY: ⚡⚡⚡⚡⚡

HOW YOU FELT AFTER EATING / SYMPTOMS:

....
....
....

DAY THREE (1 PORTION)

FLARE: YES / NO   SEVERITY: ⚡⚡⚡⚡⚡

HOW YOU FELT AFTER EATING / SYMPTOMS:

....
....
....

FOOD DIARY

-FOOD: .... REINTRODUCED ☐

START DATE: ....

DAY ONE (1/2 PORTION)

FLARE: YES / NO   SEVERITY: ⚡⚡⚡⚡⚡

HOW YOU FELT AFTER EATING / SYMPTOMS:

....

....

....

DAY TWO (3/4 PORTION)

FLARE: YES / NO   SEVERITY: ⚡⚡⚡⚡⚡

HOW YOU FELT AFTER EATING / SYMPTOMS:

....

....

....

DAY THREE (1 PORTION)

FLARE: YES / NO   SEVERITY: ⚡⚡⚡⚡⚡

HOW YOU FELT AFTER EATING / SYMPTOMS:

....

....

....

FOOD DIARY

-FOOD: .... REINTRODUCED ☐

START DATE: ....

DAY ONE (1/2 PORTION)

FLARE: YES / NO   SEVERITY: ⚡ ⚡ ⚡ ⚡ ⚡

HOW YOU FELT AFTER EATING / SYMPTOMS:

....
....
....

DAY TWO (3/4 PORTION)

FLARE: YES / NO   SEVERITY: ⚡ ⚡ ⚡ ⚡ ⚡

HOW YOU FELT AFTER EATING / SYMPTOMS:

....
....
....

DAY THREE (1 PORTION)

FLARE: YES / NO   SEVERITY: ⚡ ⚡ ⚡ ⚡ ⚡

HOW YOU FELT AFTER EATING / SYMPTOMS:

....
....
....

FOOD DIARY

-FOOD: .... REINTRODUCED ☐

START DATE: ....

DAY ONE (1/2 PORTION)

FLARE: YES / NO   SEVERITY: ⚡⚡⚡⚡⚡

HOW YOU FELT AFTER EATING / SYMPTOMS:

....
....
....

DAY TWO (3/4 PORTION)

FLARE: YES / NO   SEVERITY: ⚡⚡⚡⚡⚡

HOW YOU FELT AFTER EATING / SYMPTOMS:

....
....
....

DAY THREE (1 PORTION)

FLARE: YES / NO   SEVERITY: ⚡⚡⚡⚡⚡

HOW YOU FELT AFTER EATING / SYMPTOMS:

....
....
....

FOOD DIARY

-FOOD: .... REINTRODUCED ☐

START DATE: ....

DAY ONE (1/2 PORTION)

FLARE: YES / NO   SEVERITY: ⚡ ⚡ ⚡ ⚡ ⚡

HOW YOU FELT AFTER EATING / SYMPTOMS:

....
....
....

DAY TWO (3/4 PORTION)

FLARE: YES / NO   SEVERITY: ⚡ ⚡ ⚡ ⚡ ⚡

HOW YOU FELT AFTER EATING / SYMPTOMS:

....
....
....

DAY THREE (1 PORTION)

FLARE: YES / NO   SEVERITY: ⚡ ⚡ ⚡ ⚡ ⚡

HOW YOU FELT AFTER EATING / SYMPTOMS:

....
....
....

FOOD DIARY

-FOOD: .... REINTRODUCED ☐

START DATE: ....

DAY ONE (1/2 PORTION)

FLARE: YES / NO　　　　　　　SEVERITY: ⚡⚡⚡⚡⚡

HOW YOU FELT AFTER EATING / SYMPTOMS:

....
....
....

DAY TWO (3/4 PORTION)

FLARE: YES / NO　　　　　　　SEVERITY: ⚡⚡⚡⚡⚡

HOW YOU FELT AFTER EATING / SYMPTOMS:

....
....
....

DAY THREE (1 PORTION)

FLARE: YES / NO　　　　　　　SEVERITY: ⚡⚡⚡⚡⚡

HOW YOU FELT AFTER EATING / SYMPTOMS:

....
....
....

FOOD DIARY

-FOOD: .... REINTRODUCED ☐

START DATE: ....

DAY ONE (1/2 PORTION)

FLARE: YES / NO   SEVERITY: ⚡ ⚡ ⚡ ⚡ ⚡

HOW YOU FELT AFTER EATING / SYMPTOMS:

....
....
....

DAY TWO (3/4 PORTION)

FLARE: YES / NO   SEVERITY: ⚡ ⚡ ⚡ ⚡ ⚡

HOW YOU FELT AFTER EATING / SYMPTOMS:

....
....
....

DAY THREE (1 PORTION)

FLARE: YES / NO   SEVERITY: ⚡ ⚡ ⚡ ⚡ ⚡

HOW YOU FELT AFTER EATING / SYMPTOMS:

....
....
....

FOOD DIARY

-FOOD: .... REINTRODUCED ☐

START DATE: ....

DAY ONE (1/2 PORTION)

FLARE: YES / NO   SEVERITY: ⚡⚡⚡⚡⚡

HOW YOU FELT AFTER EATING / SYMPTOMS:

....
....
....

DAY TWO (3/4 PORTION)

FLARE: YES / NO   SEVERITY: ⚡⚡⚡⚡⚡

HOW YOU FELT AFTER EATING / SYMPTOMS:

....
....
....

DAY THREE (1 PORTION)

FLARE: YES / NO   SEVERITY: ⚡⚡⚡⚡⚡

HOW YOU FELT AFTER EATING / SYMPTOMS:

....
....
....

FOOD DIARY

-FOOD: .... REINTRODUCED ☐

START DATE: ....

DAY ONE (1/2 PORTION)

FLARE: YES / NO   SEVERITY: ⚡⚡⚡⚡⚡

HOW YOU FELT AFTER EATING / SYMPTOMS:

....
....
....

DAY TWO (3/4 PORTION)

FLARE: YES / NO   SEVERITY: ⚡⚡⚡⚡⚡

HOW YOU FELT AFTER EATING / SYMPTOMS:

....
....
....

DAY THREE (1 PORTION)

FLARE: YES / NO   SEVERITY: ⚡⚡⚡⚡⚡

HOW YOU FELT AFTER EATING / SYMPTOMS:

....
....
....

FLARES

WHILE ALL BLADDER FLARES FEEL SIMILAR, THEY ARE CAUSED BY DIFFERENT TRIGGERS. SOME OF THESE TRIGGERS INCLUDE STRESS, SEX, DIET, CLOTHING, VIBRATION, HOW LONG THE BLADDER IS HELD, HOW MUCH WATER IS DRANK AND SO ON. BEING ABLE TO IDENTIFY WHAT CAUSED THE FLARE WILL HELP YOU DETERMINE WHAT TO DO TO REDUCE THE SEVERITY AND DURATION. PLEASE KEEP IN MIND THAT NO MATTER WHAT YOU READ OR WHAT YOU HEAR ABOUT THIS PAINFUL DISORDER, YOU ARE THE ONE WHO WILL BE ABLE TO BEST IDENTIFY FLARE TYPES IN YOUR BODY. EVERY PERSON IS DIFFERENT AND YOU MAY FIND THINGS THAT WORK FOR YOU THAT DIDN'T FOR OTHERS. SO KEEP TRYING DIFFERENT THINGS UNTIL YOU TEACH YOURSELF THE TYPES OF SELF CARE THAT WILL BE BENEFICIAL TO YOU.

BLADDER WALL FLARE

THE BLADDER WALL FLARE IS GENERALLY CAUSED OR AGGRAVATED BY DIET. IT CAN FEEL MORE INTENSE WITH SOME SAYING THEY FEEL A LOT OF PRESSURE IN THE LOWER PELVIS AND/OR CLITORIS. ALL FLARES WILL BARE SIMILARITIES TO A UTI BUT BLADDER WALL FLARES MAY FEEL LESS SEVERE AFTER EMPTYING THE BLADDER.

SOME THINGS YOU CAN DO IN THIS CASE IS AN ELIMINATION DIET. RISTRICTING YOUR DIET TO THE FOODS AND BEVERAGES THAT ARE BLADDER FRIENDLY FOR YOU. FOR EXTREME FLARES DRINK PLENTY OF WATER ALL AT ONCE IN ORDER TO DILUTE THE BLADDER AND CONSUME FOODS THAT ARE ALKALINE.

PELVIC FLOOR FLARE

THE PELVIC FLOOR FLARES ARE CAUSED WHEN THE PELVIC MUSCLES GET TO TIGHT OR HAVE EXPERIENCED TRAMA. THINGS THAT CAN CAUSE OR AGGRAVATE THESE FLARES ARE SEX, A LONG CAR RIDE AND ESPECIALLY STRESS. THESE FLARES CAN FEEL DIFFERENT AS THEY MAY BE FELT IN A SLIGHTLY DIFFERENT AREA AND VARY WITH THEIR SEVERITY.

SOME THINGS YOU CAN DO IN THIS CASE ARE START STRETCHES TO LOOSEN THE PELVIC FLOOR, REDUCE STRESS, BE AWARE OF HOW YOU ARE TIGHTENING YOUR BODY WHILE STRESSED AND NOT SITTING TO LONG, TO NAME A FEW. APPLYING HEAT OR HAVING A BATH IS A GREAT WAY TO MANAGE A SEVERE PELVIC FLARE.

MUSCLE FLARE

MUSCLE FLARES CAN BE CAUSED BY MANY THINGS BUT MOST COMMONLY STRESS, CLOTHING, AND SEX. THEY CAN FEEL LESS SEVERE THEN A BLADDER WALL FLARE AND MAY BE IN A DIFFERENT LOCATION ON YOUR LOWER ABDOMEN.

TO MANAGE THESE FLARES IT CAN BE HELPFUL TO TRY DIFFERENT THINGS INCLUDING RELAXATION TECHNIQUES, HEAT AND ICE OR A WARM BATH.

SELF CARE

SELF CARE IS VERY IMPORTANT IN MANAGING YOUR IC FLARES. BELOW ARE ONLY A FEW THINGS YOU CAN TRY IN ORDER TO REDUCE THE SEVERITY AND DURATION. IF YOU CAN IDENTIFY THE TRIGGER IT WILL BE EASIER TO HELP YOURSELF FEEL BETTER. IF YOU AREN'T SURE WHAT THE TRIGGER IS THEN TRY DIFFERENT THINGS UNTIL YOU FIND SOLUTIONS THAT WORK FOR YOU.

- CONTROL YOUR DIET AND EAT LOTS OF BLADDER FRIENDLY FOODS.
- DRINK LOTS OF WATER AND KEEP YOUR BLADDER DILUTED.
- HAVE A WARM BATH.
- HEAT / ICE. TRY A HEATING PAD OR ICE PACK WHEN FLARES ARE BAD.
- SITZ BATH.
- DRINK BAKING SODA WATER IF YOU NEED URGENT RELIEF.
- PEPPERMINT CAN COOL A FLARE (TRY TEA OR MINTS).
- YOGA OR OTHER STRESS RELIEF TECNIQUES TO HELP RELAX.
- MASSAGE. YOU CAN TRY SELF MASSAGE AS WELL.
- MEDITATION.
- PH BALANCE DROPS FOR ACIDIC FOOD AND DRINKS.
- MARTIN AND PLEASANCE - BLADDER RELIEF SPRAY. THIS CAN HELP WITH SEVERE BLADDER WALL FLARES.
- WEAR COTTON UNDERWEAR.
- RELAX RELAX RELAX AND BE AWARE OF HOW YOU HOLD YOURSELF, PARTICULARLY WHERE YOU HOLD TENSION IN YOUR BODY.
- GET ENOUGH SLEEP.
- REDUCE THE STRESS IN YOUR EVERY DAY LIFE AS MUCH AS YOU CAN.
- TALK TO A UROLOGIST ABOUT TREATMENT OPTIONS SUCH AS BLADDER INSTALLMENTS OR PAIN MANAGEMENT TECNIQUES.

Made in United States
Troutdale, OR
07/08/2023